The Gift of Oriental Medicine

Written for the Western Reader:

Unwrap the Secrets That Could Heal Your Life

Anne Chew MA, MSOM, LAc, DOM

The Gift of Oriental Medicine Written for the Western Reader

Copyright © 2011 by Anne Chew

Printed in the United States of America

CONTENTS

Anne Chew MA, MSOM, LAc, DOM

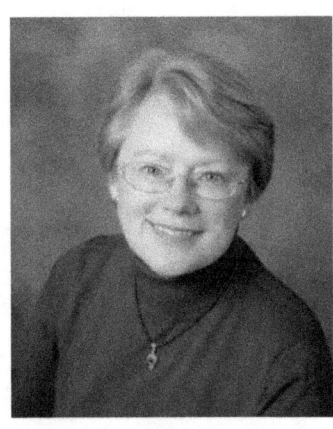

Licensed acupuncturist in the State of Colorado.

Diplomat in Acupuncture from the National Commission for Certification of Acupuncture and Oriental Medicine (NCCAOM).

Certified in Advanced Acupuncture and Moxibustion and Chinese Herbal Medicine from the China Beijing International Acupuncture Training Center.

Licensed Doctor of Oriental Medicine from the New Mexico State Board of Professional Regulation.

Education

Southwest Acupuncture College, M.S.O.M. (Master of Science in Oriental Medicine)

Florida School of Massage, Certificate in Massage and Hydrotherapy

Chapman University, M.A. in Clinical/Community Psychology

Syracuse University, B.S. in Family and Child Development and Education

The content provided in this document is for information purposes only. It is intended to provide educational material and is not designed to provide medical advice. The information may have changed in some fashion. It may be subject to debate and accuracy is not guaranteed.

Neither Anne Chew nor Acu-Choice Health Care, LLC will be held responsible regarding any medical issues relating to diseases, conditions, symptoms, diagnosis, treatment or any side effects that may arise.

The Gift of Oriental Medicine

Written for the Western Reader:

Unwrap the Secrets That Could Heal Your Life

I am using the term Oriental Medicine to include all of the Traditional Medical systems of the Far East including Chinese, Japanese, Korean and Vietnamese. The things that they have in common are that they share understanding of the body as an energetic system that can be nurtured and healed and brought into balance using lifestyle components including meditation, exercise and massage, food (nutrition), herbs, oils, acupuncture and moxibustion (moxibustion includes the burning of herbs over acupuncture points.) My primary study has been Traditional Chinese Medicine (TCM) and Japanese Acupuncture variations.

This explanation of Oriental Medicine is my interpretation of Chinese Medical concepts into a western framework that I hope will be both readable and understandable to thoughtful Westerners. My other hope is that this may help open the doors of this incredible, effective medicine to millions of suffering people who have not been able to find satisfactory help for their illnesses. Scholars of Traditional Chinese Medicine may blanch at the over-simplification of concepts. This is not written for them.

Oriental Medicine is a living organic medicine. It continues to grow and to expand utilizing new information, new discoveries and new technology as it evolves. It is traditional medicine based upon ancient wisdom and an understanding of the observed world. It is a theory of health as opposed to a theory of disease. Oriental Medicine includes a more organized and highly evolved and preserved form of herbology and natural medicine than Naturopathic medicine from Europe.

In comparing Oriental Medicine to Western Medicine it is not a matter of which is "better". Both are different ways of looking at the body each with strengths and weaknesses. If we think of the state of Colorado as the human body and a road map as Western Medicine, it works just fine if we have a car and are trying to get from Denver to Grand Junction.

It does not work well if we are trying to get to an abandoned silver mine in the mountains behind Aspen where there are no roads. Oriental Medicine works very well because it is more like a topographical map. It is helpful to know where the cliffs and waterways are as you pick a trail to the mine.

Western Medicine has many strengths. It has wonderful diagnostic technology with all the various scans that can look inside the body and identify any abnormalities. It is the medicine of choice for many acute diseases like raging infections or injuries. It is a disease model. It can provide miraculous surgeries to replace hips, repair cleft pallets and crushed bones and even replace diseased organs. It is truly the medicine of heroics.

What it does not do well is prevent disease. Nor does it deal well with sub-clinical and chronic disorders. Western Medicine's only answer is to prescribe drugs that you need to be on for the rest of your life for many common conditions such high blood pressure, depression, menstrual disorders, osteoporosis, IBS, acid reflux disease, arthritis, allergies and asthma and pain syndromes.

This is where Oriental Medicine shines. Because it is a theory of health, there are ways of identifying imbalances and treating them before they become disease. It can also treat chronic disease because it can identify and correct the underlying cause of the disease making it the original Functional Medicine. With good Oriental Medicine as primary care the need for the heroics of Western Medicine would be greatly diminished. Subsequently the astronomical costs for heroic health care could be cut substantially.

Some people are worried that Oriental Medicine is antithetical to certain religions because it has spiritual connections. Truth is truth no matter what package it comes in. It is true that Chinese Medicine has roots in Daoism which is more of a philosophy than a religion. Daoism began 2000 years before Christ walked this earth and is called "the way". Much like Native American culture it is rooted in a deep respect for the earth and the natural order of the created world.

A basic premise is that our health (spiritual, mental and physical) is to be found in harmony with the natural world. Man is said to be "Between Heaven and

Earth", both spiritual and physical. This is not very far from our modern concept, "We are spiritual beings having a physical experience."

An example: If we look at trees we see them responding to the earth's rotation to the sun. The sap or energy of the tree begins to come to the surface in the spring. By summer the leaves are in their fullness and the energy is at the surface. In fall the energy is going back in and the leaves die and fall off and by winter the energy is deep and interior. Our human energy does the same thing. It is at times of transition weather-wise and energy wise that we are most susceptible to get an infection (or a wind invasion in Chinese parlance).

That is why in TCM it is recommended that everyone get a balancing Acupuncture treatment four times a year at the change of season to balance our energy and boost immunity.

Our Christian culture would do well to incorporate this ancient wisdom/common sense into the way we structure our society and live our lives. One of the primary causes of illness in our modern society is the blatant lack of respect for our environment.

There is a great deal of evidence that we are poisoning ourselves with heavy metals, chemical exposure and altered foods. China too would do well to pay attention to its ancient wisdom and not follow the West into headlong pollution for the sake of profit.

What is currently being taught as Modern "Traditional Chinese Medicine" (TCM) has interesting roots. In 1945 the communist government saw the need for more medical services for the people. The Traditional Medicine Doctors were approached and told that if they wanted their medicine to survive then they needed to come up with a teachable body of knowledge.

Until the early twentieth century most of this traditional knowledge was passed down in families from one generation to another and was considered proprietary knowledge. There were no weekend seminars to share information. These were family secrets to be protected.

A group of prominent Traditional Doctors got together and shared information and TCM was born. A short course and a huge textbook were developed to provide thousands of "barefoot doctors" medical information so that they could care for the masses in China in the 1970's.

This information is now taught both in China and in countries around the world including the United States. Many accredited schools in the US teach a four – year course in TCM that includes a background in Western Sciences and Western diagnosis and nomenclature because there needs to be an interface with Western Medicine in our culture. Even though the amount of information that is currently available in English is staggering it is estimated that only about ten percent of the Chinese medical books have been translated for use in the West.

QI

The first concept that is very important to Chinese Medicine is the concept of QI, or Chi. QI is variously defined as spirit, life force or energy. The Chinese say that QI is produced by the organs working together. Each organ makes a part of the QI. The lung is the "Master of QI" and provides oxygen. The spleen (pancreas) and stomach provide the "nutritive QI" (nutrition) to the mix. The liver delivers the QI all over the body and nourishes the tendons and ligaments.

As Chinese Medicine was developing one of the major goals was to increase lifespan; mainly the lifespan of the emperor. To understand lifespan you have to understand Yuan QI.

Yuan QI lives between the kidneys and is said to be our heavenly inheritance including our genetics. Yuan QI is like an egg yolk. A little bit is needed every day to be the spark plug for our life force. When your Yuan QI is gone, you die. If you are living a moderate life, getting good food, adequate sleep, fresh air, exercise, feeling loved and having a purpose, at the end of any given day you will have made more QI than you have used so you begin to put a sort of an egg white around your egg yolk. This will extend your life because it will take you longer to use up your Yuan QI.

If, on the other hand you are burning the candle at both ends, having too much sex, are not getting adequate sleep or food you will burn through your Yuan QI quickly and will shorten your life. Chinese Emperors typically had many concubines and excess sex was always a concern of the Chinese Doctors who were charged with the longevity of the emperor!

13

The way powerful pharmaceutical (or recreational) drugs work according to TCM is to take a big bite out of the Yuan QI and release it quickly, thus shortening a person's life.

Channels, Meridians and Horary Clock

Channels or meridians are the pathways that the QI uses to circulate around the body much like our blood travels a predictable route throughout our arteries and veins. Acupuncture points are where the QI comes to the surface of the body. There are 365 points on twelve regular channels.

There are three yin channels starting on the chest and ending on the hands.

Lung

Heart

Pericardium

There are three yang channels starting on the hand and ending on the face. Large Intestine

Small intestine

Triple Warmer

There are three yang channels starting on the face and ending on the feet, Stomach

Bladder

Gallbladder

There are three yin channels starting on the feet and ending on the chest.

Spleen,

Kidney

Liver

It was not until the 20th century that we had sophisticated enough electrical equipment to verify that Acupuncture points were areas of greater electrical activity. Chinese theory states that the energy is concentrated in each of the twelve major bi-lateral meridians (each named after an organ) for two hours each twenty-four hour period. This is called the "horary clock" (see appendix).

An example of the usefulness of this: The clock starts at 3:00AM with the QI entering the Lung Channel. The lung channel is associated with grief. If a patient comes in saying that they wake every morning at 3:00AM and can't go back to sleep for several hours I might ask if they have allergies, asthma or unresolved grief. Many healthy people get up early in the morning and have a bowel movement. The QI is concentrated in the Large Intestine Channel between 5:00 and 7:00AM.

Organ "Energy System"

One thing that is important to note is that even though the words are the same, "liver" in a Western Medicine context is different than "Liver" in a Chinese Medicine context. In the West we look at the organ specific tissue. We might do blood tests or biopsy of that particular tissue and basically we have two options. It is either diseased or it is not.

In Chinese Medicine "liver" means the "Liver-Gallbladder Energy System" This energy system has connections all over the body. It has a huge job description that we may not recognize in the West. For example the liver is responsible for delivering energy all over the body as well as nourishing all tendons and ligaments. It is where the blood collects at night and is the seat of many emotions. It is what determines the regularity of a woman's menstrual cycle.

When the liver is stagnate and cannot deliver its energy it often pushes its energy onto its husband (the gallbladder). The gallbladder channel begins on the lateral face and goes back and forth over the head from the temples to the occipital lobes at the back of the head. This means that most tension headaches and most migraines have their root in disordered liver energy.

In the same way the Kidney Energy System in Chinese includes the entire endocrine system as we know it in the West. So thyroid, adrenal, pituitary, ovaries, testes are all part of the "Kidney-Bladder Energy System". The bottom line is that liver problems in Chinese Medicine do not equal liver disease in our

Western way of thinking. And kidney disease in Western Medicine does not equate with kidney energy problems in Chinese Medicine. The Chinese recognize when an Energy System is having difficulties long before an acute disease process shows up to alert us in Western Medicine.

Theories

Chinese Medicine is made up of many different theories that are more or less compatible. Most of them are theories of health that describe how the body works when in balance and harmony. Some of the more popular ones are:

• The need to **balance**

> ❖ yin and yang;
> ❖ QI and blood
> ❖ hot and cold
> ❖ interior and exterior
> ❖ deficiency and excess

• Channel or meridian theory explains how energy circulates around the body connecting the inside with outside. Where this energy comes to the surface is what we call acupuncture points. This energy can become stagnant just as blood and food can become stagnant. Where there is pain there is stagnant, low or blocked energy.

• Zang Fu Theory is interested in how the organs work together to provide energy to the body. These organs can become imbalanced in specific ways (not necessarily diseased in the western sense) and cause energy imbalances that account for symptoms.

The organs are put in husband and wife teams: The wife being the solid organ, the husband being the associated "empty" or "holding" organ.

The couples are:

❖ Lung & Large Intestine
❖ Spleen & Stomach
❖ Heart & Small Intestine
❖ Kidney & Bladder
❖ Liver & Gallbladder

16

If the organs are couples in a circle dance and everyone knows the dance, you have a wonderful production and flow of energy and the person feels healthy and happy. If one of the organs is having trouble with the dance, then they will bump into other organs to cause symptoms.

"Rebellious stomach QI" is a good example. If the liver energy becomes too constrained, it may "over-act" on the stomach causing the stomach QI to ascend instead of descend which is its normal direction of flow. This may cause vomiting or chronic acid reflux.

•There is a theory that explains how cold invasions (infections that are cold in nature characterized primarily by chills) enter the body and get lodged in deep energetic layers.

•There is a theory that explains how heat invasions enter the body and get stuck. This would be characterized by people who come to their doctor complaining that they had the flu six months ago (or Mono 10 years ago) and have never been really well since.

•There is a theory of how our energies change as we age. (It is different for men and women). Women primarily lose spleen or digestive energy and men lose liver energy thus women have a tendency to gain weight as they age and men tend to become more frustrated and irritable as they age. Thus the stereotypes of fat old women and grumpy old men! (See appendix)

•There is a theory on how the menstrual cycle works. The liver controls the periodicity, the spleen controls the quality and quantity of blood, the kidney controls the fertility.

•Theory of the Center says that the issue of ill health is always getting the digestion and elimination in order. The truth of this becomes more and more evident as we learn that most inflammation in the body has its origins in the gut.

•There is the Five Element Theory that has whole schools devoted to teaching only this method. This is a very interesting theory that claims to get at the deepest levels of organ energy imbalance. The Five elements are:

1. Metal (Lung & Large Intestine)

2. Water (Kidney & Bladder)

3. Wood (Liver & Gallbladder)

4. Fire (Heart & Small Intestine AND Pericardium & Triple Burner)

5. Earth (Spleen & Stomach)

These organ pairs include a solid organ and a hollow organ. They are usually referred to by the solid organ that produces the energy.

This theory has complex relationships between the organs on how they both nurture one another and how they control one another. The goal is always to BALANCE the elements. This theory also has a chart of correspondences (see appendix) that categorizes most anything you can think of as belonging to one of the elements. Two of the categories are especially interesting from a diagnostic point of view: emotions and colors.

Chinese Medicine and Emotions

Western thought has a body-mind dichotomy. Our emotions are seen separate from our body. In TCM emotions are seen as emanating from our bodies – particularly from our organs and can be useful in diagnosing what organ is out of balance.

• Lungs – grief, sorrow, depression

• Kidney – fear, phobias, anxiety

• Liver – over emotional, easily frustrated, easily irritated, easily angered, depression

• Heart – shock, anxiety, joy

• Spleen – worry, thoughtfulness

In the West we recognize Psycho-somatic – external events causing an internal response. The classic example used to be stress causing ulcers.

In TCM we recognize that the street goes both ways. Being in frustrating situations constrains the liver QI. Constrained liver QI can cause us to be more easily irritated and angered and frustrated. It doesn't take a TCM physician to see that we in America have a lot of liver imbalance.

In TCM there is only one thing that makes us sick from the "inside." There are "outside" things that make us sick. Those are "wind invasions" that include wind, heat, damp, viruses, bacteria and parasites. What is that one "inside" thing? Stuck emotions; emotions are not good, bad, right or wrong. Emotions are powerful energy that emanates from our organs that is designed to "move us". This comes from our evaluation of a situation that we find ourselves involved in.

For Example: If I should walk outside of my office and see a tiger standing in the parking lot, I would be filled with fear (if not panic) and immediately turn around, run inside my office and lock the door. The tiger's owner/trainer might have a very different response to the situation.

He might know that the tiger had eaten 50 pounds of meat that morning and was not at all hungry. He might be experiencing anxiety that someone was going to find his tiger and shoot him. Or he might be irritated that his assistant had left the door to the cage unlocked. Emotions need to be acknowledged, felt and allowed to vibrate out of us (let go of) or they will make us sick.

Skin Colors

Colors are a little more subtle but can be very helpful.

Lung: white

Kidney: black

Liver: green

Heart: red

Spleen: yellow

Ever notice how pale-white the skin of an asthmatic child often is? One time I was at a concert that was being put on by Caucasian teenage girls who were in a group home. Some were recovering from drug addiction. Drugs of any sort get their energy by taking a big bite out of our Kidney energy. Looking at them from a distance, some of the girls had an unmistakable black cast to their complexions. I'd have bet money those were the girls that had abused drugs.

Ever notice an obese red faced man that most of us would classify as a heart attack waiting to happen?

What color do we put on a hangover or nausea? Green! Alcohol is one of the hardest substances for the liver to detoxify.

Yin - Yang

Yin –Yang Chart

When yin and yang come together there is life.

When yin and yang separate there is death.

Yin	Yang
The shady side of the mountain	The sunny side of the mountain
Water	Fire
Interior	Exterior
Blood	QI
Female	Male
Dark	Light
Substance	Energy
Cold	Hot
Solid organ	Empty organ
Calm	Excited

A discussion of yin and yang is where most people's eyes begin to glaze over. How might this have anything to do with my health issues? It is a difficult concept for the westerner because we are used to thinking in terms or good vs. bad, right vs. wrong. Light is good vs. darkness is bad.

There is no value judgment with yin and yang. They are both equally valuable and necessary for life. They are concepts of comparison.

Most people would say that they prefer a sunny day (yang) (especially if they grew up in Western New York where there were long stretches of grey cloudy days (yin)). But if you live in the desert Southwest where the sun seems to always shine (yang) a rainy day (yin) is a great relief and joy. Clouds and rain bring life to the dry desert.

Most people value energy over rest. Ask an insomniac how no rest is working for them. Good rest (yin) builds good energy (yang). Most people would say that they feel great and have lots of energy the day after a good night's sleep. And people often report sleeping well after a day of vigorous exercise. They are interdependent on one another.

We need a balanced life. We need work and we need play. We need food (yin) and we need exercise (yang). **Oriental Medicine is all about moderation and balance**. Whole books have been written on the concept of yin and yang and this is just a taste of this wonderful gift.

Statements of Fact

Oriental Medicine also includes many "Statements of Fact." These are statements that explain the relationship of how things work in the body. In the West one of our statements of fact would be. "The sun rises in the east and sets in the west." No one debates whether this is true or not. We accept it at face value and take it as a working premise.

The concept of "dampness" is an important one to understand for our Western culture. Dampness includes holding water, production of excess phlegm and mucus, excess weight, and productions of tumors and masses.

One statement of fact is: "The spleen (pancreas) or digestion produces the dampness and the lung (lung, skin, throat, sinuses) is the container of the dampness." When the metabolism is in good working order there is the "arisal of the clear" meaning that we are able to take the nutrients out of the food and the "descending of the unclear" meaning that we are able to get rid of our waste products with nothing left over. If our metabolism is sluggish then we will produce dampness.

This means that there will be the arisal of the clear and the descending of the unclear and that there is turbidity (undigested, un-eliminated matter) left over. It first appears as excess fluid, phlegm, or fat. This is a profound concept for our culture when you think of all the problems with constipation, runny noses and obesity that people here deal with. Digestion and elimination are the main issues that need to be brought into balance when addressing dampness. To do that may include supporting the lung function and the kidney function as well as the spleen (digestive) function.

Another Statement of Fact says that the Kidney Energy controls the strength of the back, the strength of the knees and the hearing. This understanding is one reason that Acupuncture has gained such a good reputation in treating back pain. By treating and nourishing the "Kidney Energy" (which often means supporting the adrenal glands) (your fight or flight gland) and moving the energy to the kidney the underlying cause for the chronic back pain goes away.

Diagnosis

In TCM the primary tool for diagnosis is asking the 10 questions, which really means asking the 100 questions. An extensive questionnaire about every symptom of every system helps to point the way to an accurate diagnosis. It is the original "holistic medicine". Every symptom matters. If you have asthma your Western doctor is not interested in whether or not you have back pain. But that is crucial information to a TCM Practitioner. Asthma is not a diagnosis in TCM. It is just a symptom. The diagnosis is determining which energy patterns are out of balance.

So "wheezing' (Western diagnosis: asthma) may be caused by:

Deficiency Types

1. Weak Lung energy (can't breathe out)

2. Weak Kidney energy (can't breathe in -- kidney has to grasp the QI) (sore back)

3. Weak QI (general debility) extreme fatigue

Excess Types

1. Wind-Cold (Wind = virus, bacteria, allergen) Chills, headaches, thin white sputum

2. Heat-phlegm – (Heat = infection usually) cough with thick yellow sputum, (dampness), chest stuffiness, fever

Tongue diagnosis:

•The tongue can provide a complete map of the organs. Color, texture, coating, cracks and shape can all provide clues as to which organ is having difficulty.

Pulse diagnosis:

•Up to six pulse points can be read on each wrist for a total of twelve positions. The pulse rate and regularity are important just as in Western thought. In addition the depth, force, and quality of the pulse in each position can be diagnostic.

Remember the colors and emotions?

•Very pale face = lung, very dark facial tone = kidney.
• Sad or grieving = lung, very fearful = kidney.
Particular odors also point to specific organs as does the quality of the voice. Smelling sweet =spleen (pancreas, digestion) as does a sing-song voice.

And in truth many times actual people don't fall neatly into one category or another but are a combination of patterns.

Diagnosis involves the whole person: reading the tongue, reading the twelve pulses, asking questions, observation.

• How many times do you get up at night to go to the bathroom?
• Is your menstrual cycle regular?
• Do you have cramping?
• Do you have excessive bleeding?
• Do you sleep well?
• What time do you regularly wake up?
• Do you crave sugar?

EVERYTHING is important in TCM because it points to one energy pattern or another. And that is what is treated: an energy pattern. One herb does not fit all. It is a complete medical system. It is the original Functional Medicine and the original preventative medicine. It can be used to treat colds and infections and can often be successful in helping us avoid antibiotics. It can be helpful in reducing pain syndromes anywhere in the body.

I love it when patients come in and say that they have had all sorts of blood tests, X-rays, scans, MRI, etcetera, and everything comes back clear, and yet they still have symptoms. I know that they have come to the right place. Chinese Medicine usually has answers for the patient who comes in with a Western workup with a diagnosis that will keep them on drugs for the rest of their lives. Many times they can eliminate or drastically reduce those medications once they have balanced out the underlying causes.

- **Treatment**

Being the original holistic medicine and a theory of health, treatment is really first and foremost about patient education and life-style choices.

- **Meditation:**

The first thing that a patient must do is "meditate" according to TCM. Here in the West we might say "stress management." Or we might say that there is a recognition that a positive spiritual connection is necessary for good health.
- Who or what is the "pain in your neck?"
- What "can't you stomach?"
- Who or what is the source of your dis-ease?
- Is your body telling you that you need to make some changes?
- Do you need to forgive?

- Are there stuck emotions that need to be acknowledged and released?

- Do you need more recreation and relaxation? Where is your joy?

- **Massage:**

Tui Na (Chinese Massage) is a well developed system of massage that includes a lot of kneading type technique. It also includes stretching of the limbs and working the meridians to get more flow of QI. Massage is used extensively with small children in China. Stimulating points to support the immune system and help the body to expel infection or support organ function.

Shiatsu (Japanese Massage) is sometimes known as acupressure. This is a form of massage where the recipient remains fully clothed and lies on a mat on the floor. Shiatsu is also known as "thumb pressure". Each of the meridians is worked in the appropriate direction of flow and thumb pressure is applied to many of the acupuncture points along the meridian. The great wisdom of the Japanese is "if it hurts rub it".

- **Exercise:**

Tai QI, QI Gong (Chinese exercise)

Tai Chi is a highly structured set of poses or forms that focus on balance, flow and strength. QI Gong is a form of exercise that focuses on QI cultivation, strength and balance.

For Chinese Medicine the questions are:

Have you become too sedentary? Is it time to go to the gym, join a tai QI, yoga or Pilates class? To stretch, weight lift, walk or dance? The body was meant to move!

One statement of fact: "The spleen loves motion." How does that translate?

- Poor digestion?
- Diabetic?
- Carrying extra weight?
You need more regular exercise!

Many times when we injure a joint we quit using it. For a while that is appropriate. But then it becomes a habit. And the joint becomes stiff and immobile. Tui-Na is a combination of western massage and physical therapy to help relaxation and movement. We don't grow old and quit moving, rather we quit moving and grow old!

- **Food Therapy**

Like Hippocrates, the Father of Modern Medicine, the Chinese believe that food is our medicine. Over the centuries many specific connections to food have been observed.

For example, chicken soup is to be used when one is recovering from a cold or the flu. It has a strengthening effect on the immune system. Pears are very soothing to the gallbladder and can often calm down an irritated gallbladder.

They even had a cure for bleeding hemorrhoids. You simply needed to eat one banana a day – peel and all! Modern nutrition knows that it is the bio-flavonoids found in the white inner peel of the banana that will stop the bleeding. Modern acupuncturists are more likely to suggest taking a supplement form of the bio-flavonoids rather than eating a whole banana!

The Chinese believe that cold foods injure the spleen (digestive energy). They would counsel against cold drinks with ice and even cold salads.

Did you ever wonder why you are always served ginger with your sushi? It is for two reasons. One is because ginger is very warming to the digestion and therefore helps digestion. Second, it is because ginger is an antidote to fish poisoning.

Food Therapy advocates that we eat a wide variety of whole (unprocessed) foods – all in **moderation.** Foods, like herbs have defining tastes and therefore can be used to help or stress specific organs. Coffee for example is one of the few bitter foods in the American diet. Bitter is the taste that takes nutrients to the heart. Therefore two cups a day (not more) are recommended.

Modern nutrition is a logical extension of Chinese Food Therapy. Many Licensed Acupuncturists are excellent nutritionists who integrate ancient wisdom with modern science.

- **Acupuncture**

Acupuncture is one of Oriental Medicine's "big guns". Most Westerners think that acupuncture is what OM is all about, period. If you have read this far, YOU know better.

So how does acupuncture work? The million dollar question that every practitioner has been asked a million times!

A number of western researchers have tried to answer this question. Many theories have been put forth including the idea that the needles are stimulating the nerves or are following the bones. But in the end most researchers say that the most plausible explanation is what the Chinese say about it. That there are points on the body where the QI comes to the surface and by stimulating them you can adjust the energy flowing along the channels and thus influence the organs.

Most people are not aware that endorphins (brain chemicals associated with runner's high) were actually discovered when researchers were trying to figure out how acupuncture worked. Research in China has shown that stimulating certain points will help the body to produce more white blood cells. One thing that we know for certain is that acupuncture helps to adjust the internal pharmacy. That is one explanation for why it can be so helpful in reducing pain and calming addictions.

Remember the theory of balancing yin and yang, hot and cold and excess and deficiency? The right acupuncture treatment can do that kind of balancing very effectively. There are certain needle techniques that "tonify" energy-deficient organs and other techniques that "sedate" energy-excess organs. There are certain points on each meridian that will cool the organ and points that will drain excess energy. Sometimes points are used because of the effect on a specific organ and sometimes points are used because of their location. The upper back has a lot of Small Intestine points but they are usually used because they will release the shoulder and upper back.

Acupuncture has a cumulative effect. What that means is that one treatment builds on another. Sometimes the first treatment is a miracle. More usually the fourth or fifth is the miracle treatment because of the preceding treatments.

Some of the most effective acupuncture points are what we call "distal" points: points on the hands and feet, or points far from the location of the problem. For example: A famous point to get rid of shoulder pain is on the calf of the leg. Another method of Acupuncture involves only needling the opposite side of the problem. If your left knee hurts you would get needles on the right knee! Or your right elbow!

There are also systems of Acupuncture that involve using only the scalp, or only the ear or only the hand. You would treat the entire body from these locations. A well trained Acupuncturist has many ways to come after a problem.

In China you might get acupuncture daily for three weeks for a condition. Take two weeks off and do another three weeks. That does not fit into our cultural expectation of visiting a doctor here. Sometimes I will see a patient two or three times for the first week or two and then quickly go to once a week, or once every two weeks. More frequent visits may be necessary to break the pain pattern in the beginning.

What about the needles?

The needles are single – use (disposable), sterile, surgical stainless steel and are about the size of a human hair. They are not hypodermic needles that you get vaccinations with. Usually they can be eased into the skin so that there is no damage and minimal sensation. Most people (even those who are needle – sensitive) are so relieved once they have experienced acupuncture, that they make this treatment a regular part of their **health** care. It is hard to believe that you can become so relaxed and calm with needles in you! Calming, stress-relief is an added value to the other health benefits that the needles provide. Sometimes the needles will ache as the QI works its way through the point. One interesting phenomena is that sometimes a point will ache that does not have a needle in it! This goes away after a few minutes as the QI works through the blockage.

- **Electro-Acupuncture and laser**

Electro-acupuncture involves the use of a battery operated electrical stimulator that is hooked up to the needles to provide stronger stimulation to the points. Modern cold lasers can also be used to stimulate acupuncture points and meridians.

- **Injection Therapy**

Injection therapy does involve the use of hypodermic needles. A liquid substance (saline, homeopathic or Vitamin B-12) is injected into an acupuncture point for the purpose of providing a longer stimulation (up to 12 hours) to the particular point.

- **Magnets**

In the same way, small magnets or seeds are taped to the acupuncture points to provide on-going stimulation. You may be familiar with motion sickness wrist bands that provide stimulation to a point on the inside of the wrist (pericardium 6) to prevent motion sickness or nausea.

- **Moxibustion**

Moxibustion involves the burning of herbs (artemisia vulagaris) on specific acupuncture points for the purpose of infusing heat or yang energy into the point. There are many ways to use moxa. It can be burned directly on the skin. This is done in China but few practitioners in the US will do it because of the liability. The moxa can be balanced on the end of needles and the heat delivered through the needle. Some US practitioners do this. It can also be made into moxa rolls (they look like cigars) and held near a point that needs heat. This can be a very effective healing strategy if the issue is deficient Yang (heat) in an organ. Burning herbs in your office can create problems with other people in the building. To make matters worse, the burning Artemisia smells like marijuana. Some practitioners have signs in their office stating that the smoke smell is from moxa not pot.

I use a TDP lamp for most every treatment. It is a mineral impregnated plate that heats up and delivers penetrating warmth to the abdomen or the injured area being treated. It provides the heat without the smoke. Patients love it!

- **Cupping**

Cupping is a commonly used treatment in TCM. It is a form of suction that involves the use of glass or bamboo jars. Cotton balls are soaked in alcohol and lit on fire. The fire balls are quickly thrust in and out of the jars creating heated air in the jar. The jars are immediately placed directly on the body (usually the back). A strong suction is formed. Why would you want to do this?

Sometimes blood becomes trapped in muscle tissue. This stagnation causes aches and pain. The strong stimulation of the cupping sometimes brings the stagnant blood to the surface so the body is then able to move the blood. It is also used when there is a lot of lung congestion. The strong cupping stimulation helps to break up the congestion so the body can get rid of it.

I always ask permission before I cup someone because the treatment can leave marks on the body for up to two weeks. It looks as if you have been hugged by a giant octopus. At the very least you will have the round outline of the jars for a few days. At worst, if it has brought up a lot of stagnant blood it will take several weeks for the marks to resolve. Not something a woman wants to have to deal with if she is wearing a low cut dress for her sister's wedding.

- **Gua Sha**

Gua Sha is actually a Chinese folk remedy in that the technique is commonly used in Chinese homes. It is scraping the skin anywhere that there is pain. In China they use highly polished water buffalo horns. (Think of a tortoise shell shoe horn.) You can also use the edge of a heavy ceramic soup spoon used in Chinese restaurants. Scraping the skin where there is pain pulls energy to the area and pushes energy along the channels to get it moving. It can be used for headaches to any body ache. Sometimes the scraping will bring up Sha. Sha is the name of the stagnant blood that comes to the surface. The Sha looks like a little like dark bruising. Usually the skin just gets bright red for a few minutes from the scraping. It is a form of deep tissue massage using a tool.

- **Herbs**

Chinese Herbal Medicine is a phenomenal system of healing. It has been developed over thousands of years and continues to be refined to this day.

One major difference from our herbal use in the West is that rarely do the Chinese use a single herb by itself. Sophisticated formulas are used to treat different energy pattern disturbances.

Chinese herbs are characterized by a number of different parameters. They are classified by their taste; bitter, bland, pungent, sour, acrid, sweet and salty. They are also classified as yin or yang and hot or cold. Some herbs are said to have an affinity to specific channels (organs).

In the most comprehensive modern Materia Medica published in 1977 from Jiangsu College there are **almost 6000 entries**. It took twenty-five years to compile. A common text book for Acupuncturists in the US is "Chinese Herbal Medicine Materia Medica (revised edition)" by Bensky/Gamble. In it there are approximately **500 single herbs** that are categorized by their primary function. A few of the categories are; Herbs that Transform Phlegm and Stop Coughing, Herbs that Clear Heat and Dry Dampness, Herbs that Invigorate the Blood, Herbs that Stabilize and Bind.

In the companion textbook by the same authors "Chinese Herbal Medicine Formulas & Strategies" there are approximately **750 formulas** that are presented. These large numbers give you an idea of the breath and scope of the medicine. Many, if not most of these formulas are very old. And they work if properly prescribed. They have very few side effects because they are always **balanced.**

A balanced formula means that if an herb is used that is very cold, and therefore is damaging to the spleen (digestion) then another herb is used that will provide some gentle warmth. Most formulas have six or more herbs to provide a balanced remedy.

In Western Medicine we will often use antibiotics to fight in infection (heat invasion). Antibiotics would be classified as very cold in the Chinese classification. Many people end up with digestive problems including stomach pain and diarrhea when taking antibiotics. Antibiotics and most Western drugs are not balanced and therefore can cause unwanted side effects.

A good example of how using an herb outside of a formula can cause problems is the case of Ma Huang or Ephedra or Herba Ephedrae. When used in a Traditional Chinese Formula it is very effective in stopping wheezing and coughing. Because a small amount of it is used and it is in a balanced formula it is safe and effective without side effects. This is especially true if it is recommended for a person who has the appropriate energy pattern for the formula. However, when Ephedra is used in large amounts over a long period of time (as in weight loss formulas) it is a powerful diuretic and can cause sweating and high blood pressure as well as insomnia, heart arrhythmias and tremors. It can be very dangerous used in this way.

Fire can destroy a city or a forest yet when used in a controlled manner like the burning of propane to heat your house it is a modern wonder. To ban the use of fire because of forest fires would be a real loss to humankind. Banning the use of certain herbs because untrained people have abused them is an equal loss to humankind.

What does Oriental Medicine treat?

Oriental Medicine is a **complete medical system** that can treat most emotional and internal medical concerns including but not limited to: headaches of all kinds, digestive issues of all kinds, menstrual irregularities, menopause, allergies, weight issues, asthma-type symptoms, bladder issues, parasites, sinus issues, high and low blood pressure, high cholesterol, high and low blood sugar, depression, anxiety, PMS, GERD, high liver enzymes, auto-immune disorders, thyroid and adrenal problems, fatigue, insomnia, etc..

It can treat all muscular-skeletal pain syndromes such as: back pain of all kinds, shoulder pain, hip pain, knee pain, postsurgical pain, injuries of all kinds, fibromyalgia, arthritis pain, neck pain….you get the idea, anything that includes pain.

It can treat infectious disease especially in the early stages and if the disease becomes chronic (you just cannot get rid of it). Often you can avoid the use of an antibiotic by using Oriental Medicine. Sometimes it is appropriate to use both medicines if you have cooperating, knowledgeable practitioners.

What does it not treat?

Oriental Medicine does not treat broken bones, except after the bone has been set. Oriental Medicine does not do anything surgical, or prescribe controlled pharmaceutical drugs.

Western Medicine is fantastic at diagnosis with X-rays, MRI, CAT scans, ultrasound, sophisticated blood analysis, etcetera. I often send my patients to their MD's or DO's to have these tests when I suspect a problem that needs more clarification. If Western diagnostic tools uncover a problem that I can treat and that is what the patient wants, then that is the direction we go. Sometimes Western treatment is more appropriate and I will encourage and support that.

In China, both medicines are practiced side-by-side. They are looking to find what modality treats what problems the best. Stroke victims are treated first with Western Medicine then immediately sent to the Acupuncture clinic (in the hospital) for ongoing therapy. Cancer patients are treated with chemo and immediately (the same day) sent to Acupuncture to mitigate the side effects. This is a model that could save billions of dollars if adopted in the West.

During my study in Beijing I sat with a Chinese TCM Doctor who would listen to a patient's complaints, ask questions, take the pulse, look at the tongue and then order blood tests and basic scans (ultrasounds or x-rays) as needed. The patient would walk down the hall to the lab, get the needed tests and then return with the results. With this expanded information the doctor would then prescribe the appropriate herbal formulas.

Education and NCCAOM

One good way of finding someone fully qualified to do acupuncture is to visit the website for the **National Certification Commission for Acupuncture and Oriental Medicine.** Most states require that persons be diplomats and certified by the NCCAOM (which includes high educational standards and national examination) in order to be licensed as Acupuncturists. Standards for acupuncture include a minimum of 1905 hours of training including 660 hours of clinic training. This minimum would take three years to complete. Many schools are four years of study. Looking for State Licensed Acupuncturists is another way of finding someone who is fully qualified.

You need be aware that because this is such a new profession in the United States when the laws regulating the practice of Acupuncture were written, other professions (Medical Doctors and Chiropractors) that have more political clout (money) made sure that acupuncture was included in their scope of practice. Often very brief courses of study are all that are required for them to practice. Some states are allowing physical therapists to take a weekend course and to do "dry needling". (Acupuncture by another name.)

Acupuncture and Oriental Medicine is very powerful medicine. Over half the world's population uses it. It is also very safe for well trained persons to do it. The proof of that is that mal-practice insurance is very inexpensive because there are so few claims made against practitioners. (First,…do no harm…) Make sure you are getting the best that Oriental Medicine has to offer you and see a fully qualified person.

Summary

Oriental Medicine is an exciting primary **HEATH CARE** model that brings the best of traditional wisdom to modern health concerns. **It is holistic, safe, effective, preventative and gets to the root of the problem (functional).** It has thousands of years of proven effectiveness behind it.

Most people would benefit from having a qualified Oriental Medicine Practitioner on their health care team.

If insurance companies were informed and smart they could save themselves and their customers time, money, pain and suffering by providing Acupuncture and Oriental Medical Benefits.

Appendices

Five Element Correspondence Chart

Element	Wood	Fire	Earth	Metal	Water
Yin	Liver	Heart	Spleen	Lung	Kidney
Yang	Gallbladder	Small Intestine	Stomach	Large Intestine	Bladder
Emotion	Anger, irritation, over-emotional, frustration	Joy, Shock	Desire, pensiveness, worry	Grief	Fear
Flavor	Sour	Bitter	Sweet	Pungent & spicy	Salty
Season	Spring	Summer	Late Summer	Autumn	Winter
Sense	Vision	Speech	Taste	Smell	Hearing
Orifice	Eyes	Tongue	Mouth	Nose	Ears
Color	Green	Red	Yellow	White	Black
Sounds	Shouting	Laughing	Singing	Weeping	Groaning

The QI Cycle for Men

Age 8	The Kidney QI becomes abundant, the hair begins to grow longer, the teeth begin to change
Age 16	The Kidney QI becomes more abundant, he begins to have his heaven cycle, he is full of (semen), he can ejaculate and have a child, and intercourse is possible.
Age 24	The Kidney QI is equal (i.e. Kidney yin-yang are balanced), the tendons, muscles, bones become strong, the wisdom teeth grow
Age 32	All tendons, muscles, bones in top condition (you are at the top of your game!)
Age 40	The Kidney QI weakens, the hair begins to fall off, the teeth begin to wither
Age 48	The Yang QI in the upper part of the body declines with the complexion looking withered, hair turns grey
Age 56	The Liver QI begins to weaken, the heaven cycle becomes exhausted, the jing (semen) becomes scanty, the kidney organs decline, all parts of the body begin to grow old
Age 64	All hair and teeth are gone (Yikes!)

The QI Cycle for Women

Age 7	Kidney QI becomes abundant, the hair begins to grow longer, the teeth begin to change
Age 14	The Ren mai begins to flow, the "heaven cycle" begins, the Chong Mai begins to grow in abundance, menstruation begins, pregnancy is possible
Age 21	The Kidney QI becomes equal (i.e. the yin-yang are balanced), the wisdom teeth begin to grow
Age 28	The tendons, muscles, bones become hard, the hair grows to the longest, the body and mind are in top condition
Age 35	The yang ming meridians begin to weaken with the result that the complexion starts to wither, the hair begins to fall off
Age 42	The 3 yang meridians of the hands and legs begin to weaken, the complexion looks even more withered, the hair turns grey
Age 49	The Ren mai becomes deficient, the heaven cycle becomes exhausted, the Chong mai becomes weakened and scanty, her body becomes old, she can't become pregnant

The Horary Clock

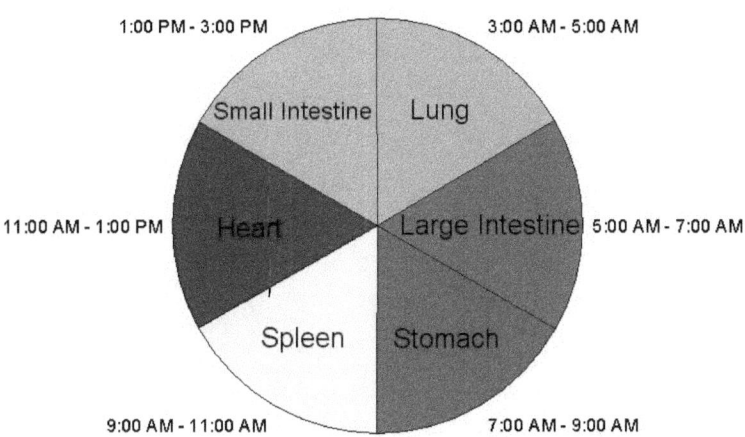

The Horary Clock

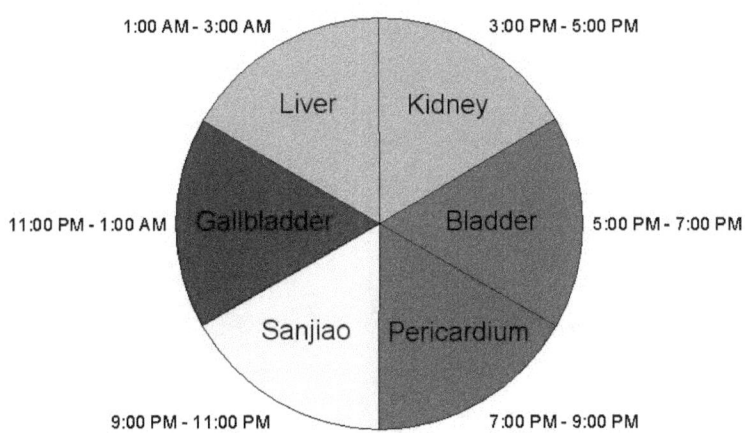

Personal Notes:

ABOUT ACU-CHOICE HEALTH CARE

Sometimes, conventional medicine fails to bring us lasting relief. Anne Chew, MA, MSOM, LAc, DOM, Founder of Acu-Choice Health Care, has had this experience personally and understands your desire for health and well-being. As a result, she works with you to develop a personalized treatment plan, designed to guide you toward a lifetime of wellness. This unique approach includes an evaluation from a Traditional Chinese Medicine perspective, a dietary review, lab tests such as food allergy, and saliva hormone panels and a treatment plan. Treatments usually include:

•A lifetime dietary plan.
•Nutritional supplements including vitamins, minerals and herbs. Some recommendations are short term to clear a condition and others are long term for prevention.
•Acupuncture for re-balancing the organ-energy systems and pain relief.
•Clearing of emotional and word patterns when necessary.
•Detoxification testing and treatment, including ionic foot baths when necessary.

Visit our website at http://www.acuchoice.net
Email us for more information about Acu-Choice. acuchoice@yahoo.com

Acu-Choice Health Care
3470 South Sherman Street #1
Englewood, Colorado 80113
Phone: 303-794-9505
Fax: 303-736-6767

Follow Acu-Choice Health Care on Twitter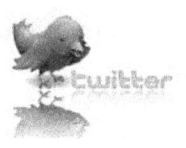

http://twitter.com/Acuchoice

Read our blog WORDPRESS *http://acuchoice.wordpress.com/*

Find us on Facebook 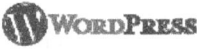 *http://www.facebook.com/people/Anne-Chew/100001443332164*

Read Anne's articles at **Ezine** *@rticles*

http://ezinearticles.com/?expert=Anne_Chew

www.ingramcontent.com/pod-product-compliance
Lightning Source LLC
Chambersburg PA
CBHW071730170526
45165CB00005B/2224